SUMMA

EVALUATION OF

PEPFAR

Committee on the Outcome and Impact Evaluation of Global HIV/AIDS Programs Implemented Under the Lantos-Hyde Act of 2008

Board on Global Health
Board on Children, Youth, and Families

INSTITUTE OF MEDICINE
OF THE NATIONAL ACADEMIES

THE NATIONAL ACADEMIES PRESS
Washington, D.C.
www.nap.edu

THE NATIONAL ACADEMIES PRESS 500 Fifth Street, NW Washington, DC 20001

NOTICE: The project that is the subject of this report was approved by the Governing Board of the National Research Council, whose members are drawn from the councils of the National Academy of Sciences, the National Academy of Engineering, and the Institute of Medicine. The members of the committee responsible for the report were chosen for their special competences and with regard for appropriate balance.

This study was supported by Contract/Grant No. SAQMMA09M0693 between the National Academy of Sciences and the U.S. Department of State. Any opinions, findings, conclusions, or recommendations expressed in this publication are those of the author(s) and do not necessarily reflect the views of the organizations or agencies that provided support for the project.

International Standard Book Number-13: 978-0-309-26780-9
International Standard Book Number-10: 0-309-26780-3
Library of Congress Control Number: 2013939517

Additional copies of this Summary are available in limited quantities from the Institute of Medicine, 500 Fifth Street, NW, Washington, DC 20001.

Copies of *Evaluation of PEPFAR*, from which this Summary has been extracted, are available for sale from the National Academies Press, 500 Fifth Street, NW, Keck 360, Washington, DC 20001; (800) 624-6242 or (202) 334-3313; http://www.nap.edu.

For more information about the Institute of Medicine, visit the IOM home page at: **www.iom.edu.**

Printed in the United States of America

The serpent has been a symbol of long life, healing, and knowledge among almost all cultures and religions since the beginning of recorded history. The serpent adopted as a logotype by the Institute of Medicine is a relief carving from ancient Greece, now held by the Staatliche Museen in Berlin.

Suggested citation: IOM (Institute of Medicine). 2013. *Evaluation of PEPFAR*. Washington, DC: The National Academies Press.

"Knowing is not enough; we must apply.
Willing is not enough; we must do."
—Goethe

INSTITUTE OF MEDICINE
OF THE NATIONAL ACADEMIES

Advising the Nation. Improving Health.

THE NATIONAL ACADEMIES

Advisers to the Nation on Science, Engineering, and Medicine

The **National Academy of Sciences** is a private, nonprofit, self-perpetuating society of distinguished scholars engaged in scientific and engineering research, dedicated to the furtherance of science and technology and to their use for the general welfare. Upon the authority of the charter granted to it by the Congress in 1863, the Academy has a mandate that requires it to advise the federal government on scientific and technical matters. Dr. Ralph J. Cicerone is president of the National Academy of Sciences.

The **National Academy of Engineering** was established in 1964, under the charter of the National Academy of Sciences, as a parallel organization of outstanding engineers. It is autonomous in its administration and in the selection of its members, sharing with the National Academy of Sciences the responsibility for advising the federal government. The National Academy of Engineering also sponsors engineering programs aimed at meeting national needs, encourages education and research, and recognizes the superior achievements of engineers. Dr. Charles M. Vest is president of the National Academy of Engineering.

The **Institute of Medicine** was established in 1970 by the National Academy of Sciences to secure the services of eminent members of appropriate professions in the examination of policy matters pertaining to the health of the public. The Institute acts under the responsibility given to the National Academy of Sciences by its congressional charter to be an adviser to the federal government and, upon its own initiative, to identify issues of medical care, research, and education. Dr. Harvey V. Fineberg is president of the Institute of Medicine.

The **National Research Council** was organized by the National Academy of Sciences in 1916 to associate the broad community of science and technology with the Academy's purposes of furthering knowledge and advising the federal government. Functioning in accordance with general policies determined by the Academy, the Council has become the principal operating agency of both the National Academy of Sciences and the National Academy of Engineering in providing services to the government, the public, and the scientific and engineering communities. The Council is administered jointly by both Academies and the Institute of Medicine. Dr. Ralph J. Cicerone and Dr. Charles M. Vest are chair and vice chair, respectively, of the National Research Council.

www.national-academies.org

COMMITTEE ON THE OUTCOME AND IMPACT EVALUATION OF GLOBAL HIV/AIDS PROGRAMS IMPLEMENTED UNDER THE LANTOS-HYDE ACT OF 2008

ROBERT E. BLACK (*Chair*), Johns Hopkins University, Baltimore, MD
JUDITH D. AUERBACH, Consultant, San Francisco AIDS Foundation, CA
MARY T. BASSETT, Doris Duke Charitable Foundation, New York, NY
RONALD BROOKMEYER, University of California, Los Angeles
LOLA DARE, Center for Health Sciences Training, Research and Development International, Ibadan, Nigeria
ALEX C. EZEH, African Population and Health Research Center, Nairobi, Kenya
SOFIA GRUSKIN, University of Southern California, Los Angeles
ANGELINA KAKOOZA, Makerere University College of Health Sciences, Kampala, Uganda
JENNIFER KATES, Henry J. Kaiser Family Foundation, Washington, DC
ANN KURTH, New York University, New York
ANNE C. PETERSEN, University of Michigan and Global Philanthropy Alliance, Ann Arbor
DOUGLAS D. RICHMAN, VA San Diego Healthcare System and University of California, San Diego
JENNIFER PRAH RUGER, Yale University, New Haven, CT
DEBORAH L. RUGG, United Nations Inspection and Evaluation Division, New York, NY
DAWN K. SMITH, U.S. Centers for Disease Control and Prevention, Atlanta, GA
PAPA SALIF SOW, Bill & Melinda Gates Foundation, Seattle, WA
SALLY K. STANSFIELD,[1] Independent Consultant, Geneva, Switzerland
TAHA E. TAHA, Johns Hopkins University, Baltimore, MD
KATHRYN WHETTEN, Duke University, Durham, NC
CATHERINE M. WILFERT, Retired, Elizabeth Glaser Pediatric AIDS Foundation, Durham, NC

Consultants

SHARON KNIGHT, East Carolina University, Greenville, NC
KATHRYN TUCKER, Statistics Collaborative, Inc., Washington, DC
JANET WITTES, Statistics Collaborative, Inc., Washington, DC

[1] Committee member through August 2012.

Staff

KIMBERLY A. SCOTT, Study Co-Director
BRIDGET B. KELLY, Study Co-Director
MARGARET HAWTHORNE, Program Officer
LIVIA NAVON, Program Officer
CARMEN CECILIA MUNDACA, Postdoctoral Fellow
IJEOMA EMENANJO, Senior Program Associate (through January 2011)
MILA C. GONZÁLEZ DÁVILA, Associate Program Officer (through August 2012)
KRISTEN DANFORTH, Research Associate
REBECCA MARKSAMER, Research Associate (from August 2012)
KATE MECK, Research Associate
COLLIN WEINBERGER, Research Associate (April 2011 through June 2012)
LEIGH CARROLL, Research Assistant (from October 2011)
TESSA BURKE, Senior Program Assistant (through May 2011)
ANGELA CHRISTIAN, Program Associate
WENDY E. KEENAN, Program Associate
JULIE WILTSHIRE, Financial Associate
KIMBER BOGARD, Board Director, Board on Children, Youth, and Families (from October 2011)
ROSEMARY CHALK, Board Director, Board on Children, Youth, and Families (through July 2011)
PATRICK KELLEY, Senior Board Director, Boards on Global Health and African Science Academy Development

Reviewers

This report has been reviewed in draft form by individuals chosen for their diverse perspectives and technical expertise, in accordance with procedures approved by the National Research Council's Report Review Committee. The purpose of this independent review is to provide candid and critical comments that will assist the institution in making its published report as sound as possible and to ensure that the report meets institutional standards for objectivity, evidence, and responsiveness to the study charge. The review comments and draft manuscript remain confidential to protect the integrity of the deliberative process. We wish to thank the following individuals for their review of this report:

PIERRE BARKER, Institute for Healthcare Improvement
CHRIS BEYRER, Johns Hopkins University
ANASTASIA TZAVARAS CATSAMBAS, EnCompass LLC
DAVID CELENTANO, Johns Hopkins University
PAUL DE LAY, Joint United Nations Programme on HIV/AIDS
WAFAA M. EL-SADR, Columbia University
KURT FIRNHABER, Right to Care
MITCHELL H. GAIL, National Institutes of Health
ROBERT GROSS, University of Pennsylvania
JOHN E. LANGE, Bill & Melinda Gates Foundation
CHEWE LUO, United Nations Children's Fund
JONATHON LEE SIMON, Boston University
RJ SIMONDS, Elizabeth Glaser Pediatric AIDS Foundation

SHOSHANNA SOFAER, City University of New York
MIRIAM WERE, University of Nairobi

Although the reviewers listed above have provided many constructive comments and suggestions, they were not asked to endorse the conclusions or recommendations, nor did they see the final draft of the report before its release. The review of this report was overseen by **Kristine M. Gebbie**, Flinders University School of Nursing and Midwifery, and **Ann M. Arvin**, Stanford University. Appointed by the National Research Council and Institute of Medicine, they were responsible for making certain that an independent examination of this report was carried out in accordance with institutional procedures and that all review comments were carefully considered. Responsibility for the final content of this report rests entirely with the authoring committee and the institution.

Acknowledgments

The committee, project staff, and consultants are deeply appreciative of the diverse and valuable contributions made by so many who assisted with this study.

For information and support provided throughout the project, we thank the staff of the Office of the U.S. Global AIDS Coordinator, with particular gratitude to Paul Bouey and Tiffany Parker, who facilitated our engagement during the study, as well as staff from other President's Emergency Plan for AIDS Relief (PEPFAR) implementing agencies. We are also grateful to the leadership of the U.S. missions and the PEPFAR staff in the countries visited for this evaluation, whose hospitable and gracious assistance was essential to the success of our country visits. We also thank the many other individuals in the countries visited who assisted us with logistics and support during our visits.

We are grateful to Eran Bendavid from Stanford University for his valuable consultation during the study. We appreciate the essential technical support provided to the project by Danielle Beaulieu, Jessica Case, Megan Somerday, Jeff Steen, and Neil Wohlford from Statistics Collaborative, Inc. We thank Kathryn Stadeli from University of California, San Diego, School of Medicine for her assistance with research for the study. We also thank Megan Perez and Meredith Cantwell for their excellent work on this study as interns at the Institute of Medicine as well as Wyatt Smith and Peter Dull, who provided temporary assistance during the project. We are grateful to Teresa Bergen and Diane Wellman for their diligent work as transcriptionists. We appreciate the creativity and effort of Jay Christian and LeAnn Locher for their design work. In addition, we convey our deep gratitude and appreciation for the hard work of the many staff in various offices of the Institute of Medicine and the National Academies who lent their support to the project.

There are a number of other individuals who were crucial for the administrative and logistical success of this project. For help with scheduling and communication for the committee, we thank Sharon Abbruscato, Lola Adedokun, Philomena Agaloi, Jillian Albertolli, Michele Augustus, Nkiru Azikiwe, Anna Both, Cindy Chu, Kyle Hamilton, Jennifer Heflin, Maria Male, Sheila Mwero, Catherine Nyawire, Audrey Palix, Jessica Raback, Mary Rybczynski, Fortuna Salinas, Abir Shady, Cassie Toner, Rachel Upton, Kevin Vavasseur, Jackylene Wegoki, and Marie Young. We are also immensely grateful to Anthony Mavrogiannis and the staff at Kentlands Travel for their assistance with the complex travel needs of this project.

Finally, although we cannot name them here for reasons of confidentiality, we offer our most profound thanks to the hundreds of individuals who participated in interviews and site visits as part of the evaluation data collection effort. Their generosity with their time and their willingness to share their insights were fundamental to the evaluation; it was a privilege and an inspiration to hear directly from those whose dedication and tremendous effort underlie the successes of the response to HIV globally and in PEPFAR partner countries.

Contents

The contents of the entire report, from which this Summary and the chapters' Main Messages are extracted, are listed below.

PART IV: FUTURE OF U.S. GOVERNMENT INVOLVEMENT IN THE GLOBAL RESPONSE TO HIV/AIDS

Tables, Figures, and Boxes

TABLES

FIGURES

BOXES

Preface

The HIV/AIDS pandemic has beleaguered the world for more than three decades. The countries most affected continue to be in sub-Saharan Africa, home to an estimated two-thirds of people living with HIV. There have been major increases in international aid assistance as well as in national commitments to and investments in HIV prevention, treatment, care, and capacity building activities, yet funding remains insufficient to meet the estimated immediate and projected needs.

In 2003, in response to the devastating consequences of the HIV pandemic, the U.S. Congress funded a major new U.S. global health initiative, which became known as the President's Emergency Plan for AIDS Relief, or PEPFAR.[1] PEPFAR remains the largest bilateral initiative aimed at addressing HIV/AIDS. At the time of its initial authorization, PEPFAR was seen as a bold initiative, testing, among other strategies, whether treatment could be successfully and intensively scaled up in low-resource settings. The initial authorizing language mandated that the Institute of Medicine (IOM) assess the progress of PEPFAR implementation to help guide the future directions of this innovative program. The findings and recommendations of that IOM study, published in 2007, informed PEPFAR processes, policies, and activi-

[1] United States Leadership Against HIV/AIDS, Tuberculosis, and Malaria Act of 2003, P.L. 108-25, 108th Cong., 1st sess. (May 27, 2003).

ties as well as the legislation that reauthorized the initiative, known as the Lantos-Hyde Act of 2008.[2]

The reauthorization legislation mandated that the IOM assess the performance of U.S.-assisted global HIV/AIDS programs and evaluate the impact on health of prevention, treatment, and care efforts supported by U.S. funding (see Appendix A for the statement of task). This report is intended to provide a rigorous, evidence-based, multidisciplinary, and independent evaluation of PEPFAR to Congress and the Department of State as well as to the scientific community, program implementers, policy makers, civil society, people living with and affected by HIV/AIDS, and international stakeholders in global public health.

In response to its mandate, IOM first convened a planning committee to develop a strategic approach for conducting the evaluation. This approach, published in a 2010 report, addressed the complexities of evaluating an initiative with the scale and diversity of programs that PEPFAR supports and with the range of countries in which it operates. The dynamism of an initiative that was operating and evolving over the course of the evaluation presented additional complexity.

To carry out the evaluation, the IOM convened a diverse expert committee that included considerable overlap with the members of the planning committee. Guided by the strategic approach, the committee, IOM staff, and consultants carried out a mixed-methods approach. The qualitative data that were collected included extensive document review and more than 400 semi-structured interviews conducted from 2010 to 2012. Each member of the committee visited at least one PEPFAR partner country, and in total the evaluation team conducted 13 data collection visits to partner countries, hearing the perspectives of a wide range of stakeholders. PEPFAR headquarters and mission staff, partner country stakeholders, and global partners all generously contributed their time and experience to the committee. Quantitative data included financial data, program and clinical monitoring data, and epidemiological information. The committee struggled to find quantitative data to address some of the elements of the statement of task. Beyond the specific issues of available data to address the legislated task, however, there is also the critical imperative that PEPFAR be able to determine the key questions to ask in order to assess its own performance and effectiveness and to plan in advance for the collection of meaningful data to answer those questions and guide the ongoing evolution of PEPFAR.

---

[2] Tom Lantos and Henry J. Hyde United States Global Leadership Against HIV/AIDS, Tuberculosis, and Malaria Reauthorization Act of 2008, P.L. 110-293, 110th Cong., 2nd sess. (July 30, 2008).

The 2008 reauthorization of PEPFAR emphasized that the program must transition from its initial goal of providing an emergency response to longer-term goals of enhancing sustainability, promoting country ownership, and strengthening health systems. One of the clear findings that emerged from this evaluation is that as PEPFAR evolves in this way, major dilemmas are emerging that create tensions for decision making related to a country's HIV response; these dilemmas will require attention as the program moves forward. As the HIV response becomes more country-driven, PEPFAR—and any other external donor effort—will need to focus its contributions on national efforts rather than on the direct provision of services and attribution of results. This will have consequences for program planning, implementation, and evaluation. Furthermore, focusing on country ownership will require relinquishing some control over the response, which in turn will have unknown consequences for quality and access to services; PEPFAR and its partner countries will have to grapple with these issues together.

PEPFAR has been globally transformative—changing in many ways the paradigm of global health and what can be accomplished with ambitious goals, ample funding, and humanitarian commitment to a public health crisis. As it moves forward, PEPFAR must continue to be bold in its vision, implementation, and global leadership, but now toward its aims of continuing to strengthen the capacity of partner countries to respond to the pandemic. The committee hopes that this evaluation will serve as a tool to achieve these aims.

The committee extends its gratitude to all those who provided information to assist in the evaluation. The committee has continuing deep admiration for those carrying out the difficult work of responding to the pandemic. I was privileged to serve as the chair for both the planning committee and the evaluation committee. I would like to express my appreciation to the members of both committees for the expertise and perspective they contributed, for their robust participation in discourse and deliberation, and for the immeasurable time and energy they volunteered. The IOM committee staff, very ably led by study co directors Bridget Kelly and Kimberly Scott, have been highly professional, thoughtful, and committed to ensuring the most responsive and rigorous evaluation possible. I thank the entire staff and the committee consultants for their tireless efforts in support of the committee.

Robert E. Black, *Chair*
Committee on the Outcome and Impact Evaluation of Global
HIV/AIDS Programs Implemented Under the Lantos-Hyde Act of 2008

Acronyms and Abbreviations

AIDS	acquired immune deficiency syndrome
ANC	antenatal care
APR	annual program results
ART	antiretroviral therapy
ARV	antiretroviral
AZT	zidovudine
BCC	behavior change communication
BPE	basic program evaluation
CBO	community-based organization
CCM	country coordinating mechanism
CD4	cluster of differentiation 4
CDC	U.S. Centers for Disease Control and Prevention
CGD	Center for Global Development
CHERG	Child Health Epidemiology Reference Group
CHSW	community health or para-social worker
COP	country operational plan
COPRS	Country Operational Plan Reporting System
CPT	cotrimoxazole preventive therapy
CRC	Committee on the Rights of the Child
CSO	civil society organization
CTX	cotrimoxazole

DAH development assistance for health
DHAP Division of HIV/AIDS Prevention (at CDC)
DHS Demographic and Health Surveys
DoD U.S. Department of Defense
DoL U.S. Department of Labor
DoS U.S. Department of State

EA expenditure analysis
EID early infant diagnosis of HIV

FBO faith-based organization
FELTP Field Epidemiology and Laboratory Training Program
FETP Field Epidemiology Training Program
FY fiscal year

GAO U.S. Government Accountability Office
GBV gender-based violence
GHI U.S. Global Health Initiative
Global Fund Global Fund to Fight AIDS, Tuberculosis, and Malaria
GMS Grants Management Solutions
GNI gross national income

HAPSAT HIV/AIDS Program Sustainability Analysis Tool
HHS U.S. Department of Health and Human Services
HIPC heavily indebted poor country
HIS health information system
HIV human immunodeficiency virus
HMIS health management information system
HQ headquarters
HRH human resources for health
HRSA Health Resources and Services Administration
HSS health systems strengthening

IeDEA International Epidemiological Database to Evaluate AIDS
IGA income-generating activity
IOM Institute of Medicine
IPT isoniazid preventive therapy
IPTp intermittent preventive treatment of malaria for pregnant women
ITN insecticide-treated net

LIMS laboratory information management system
LTFu loss to follow-up

M&E	monitoring and evaluation
MAT	medication-assisted treatment
MCC	Millennium Challenge Corporation
MCH	maternal and child health
MDG	Millennium Development Goal
MEPI	Medical Education Partnership Initiative
MERG	Monitoring and Evaluation Reference Group
MICS	Multiple Indicator Cluster Survey
MOH	ministry of health
MSM	men who have sex with men
MTCT	mother-to-child transmission
NAC	National AIDS Commission/Committee/Council/Control Agency
NAS	National Academies of Science
NASA	national AIDS spending assessment
NDOH	National Department of Health (South Africa)
NEPI	Nursing/Midwifery Education Partnership Initiative
NGI	next generation indicator
NGO	nongovernmental organization
NHA	national health account
NIH	U.S. National Institutes of Health
NRC	National Research Council
NSF	National Science Foundation
OECD	Organisation for Economic Co-operation and Development
OGAC	Office of the U.S. Global AIDS Coordinator
OI	opportunistic infection
OMB	Office of Management and Budget
OVC	orphans and vulnerable children
PCR	polymerase chain reaction
PEP	post-exposure prophylaxis
PEPFAR	The President's Emergency Plan for AIDS Relief
PEPFAR I	The President's Emergency Plan for AIDS Relief (2004–2008)
PEPFAR II	The President's Emergency Plan for AIDS Relief (2009–2013)
PEQ	priority evaluation question
PF	Partnership Framework
PFIP	Partnership Framework implementation plan
PHE	public health evaluation

PI	principal investigator
PICT	provider-initiated counseling and testing
PIP	Program Impact Pathway
PLHIV	people living with HIV/AIDS
PMI	President's Malaria Initiative
PMTCT	prevention of mother-to-child transmission
PPP	public–private partnership
PrEP	pre-exposure prophylaxis
QA	quality assurance
QI	quality improvement
RFA	request for application
SAB	Scientific Advisory Board (of PEPFAR)
SAMHSA	Substance Abuse and Mental Health Services Administration
SANAC	South African National AIDS Council
SAPR	semi-annual program results
SCMS	Supply Chain Management System
SGBV	sexual and gender-based violence
SI	strategic information
SOPA	State of the Program Area
STD	sexually transmitted disease
STI	sexually transmitted infection
TA	technical assistance
TAB	technical advisory board
TB	tuberculosis
TDR	transmitted drug resistance
TE	targeted evaluation
TWG	technical working group
UN	United Nations
UNAIDS	Joint United Nations Programme on HIV/AIDS
UNGASS	United Nations General Assembly Special Session
UNICEF	United Nations Children's Fund
UNODC	United Nations Office on Drugs and Crime
USAID	United States Agency for International Development
USG	U.S. government
VMMC	voluntary medical male circumcision
WHO	World Health Organization

INTERVIEW CITATION ABBREVIATIONS

Country Visit Exit Synthesis: Country # + ES
Country Visit Interview: Country # + Interview # + Organization Type
Non-Country Visit Interview: "NCV" + Interview # + Organization Type

Organization Types

USG	U.S. government
USNGO	U.S. nongovernmental organization
USPS	U.S. private sector
USACA	U.S. academia
PCGOV	partner country government
PCNGO	partner country nongovernmental organization
PCPS	partner country private sector
PCACA	partner country academia
CCM	country coordinating mechanism
ML	multilateral organization
OBL	other (non-U.S. and non-partner country) bilateral
OGOV	other government
ONGO	other (non-U.S. and non-partner country) nongovernmental organization

Summary

The U.S. government supports global HIV programs through an initiative known as the President's Emergency Plan for AIDS Relief (PEPFAR).[1] As the largest donor to the global response to HIV, the U.S. government is making an historic contribution, benefitting in particular countries that have limited available resources and infrastructure and a great need for support of their national responses to HIV.

PEPFAR is a large, multifaceted, and complex initiative that is implemented in the cultural, social, economic, and political landscapes of each partner country as well as in the presence of HIV and health programs supported by other funding sources. Working through many implementing partners, PEPFAR supports a range of activities for all aspects of the HIV response, including direct service provision, programmatic support, technical assistance, and policy facilitation.

In light of the magnitude of the HIV crisis at the time, PEPFAR initially focused on the urgent need to scale up HIV services, accompanied by expectations for accountability and performance measurement. In addition, the authorizing legislation recognized the need for a long-term, comprehensive, international response. PEPFAR has achieved—and in some

[1] PEPFAR was authorized by the U.S. Congress in two phases: PEPFAR I (FY 2004–FY 2008) in the United States Leadership Against HIV/AIDS, Tuberculosis, and Malaria Act of 2003 (P.L. 108-25) and PEPFAR II (FY 2009–FY 2013) in the Tom Lantos and Henry J. Hyde United States Global Leadership Against HIV/AIDS, Tuberculosis, and Malaria Reauthorization Act of 2008 (P.L. 110-293).

cases surpassed—its initial ambitious aims. These efforts have saved and improved the lives of millions of people around the world. That success has in effect "reset" the baseline and shifted global expectations for what can be achieved in partner countries. The reauthorization of PEPFAR not only set new aims to continue to scale up services, but also heightened the emphasis on health systems strengthening and sustainability, a shift in focus that has been increasingly reflected in the initiative's policies, activities, and dialogue with stakeholders.

EVALUATION APPROACH

The statement of task for this evaluation was derived from the legislation that reauthorized PEPFAR, which mandated that the Institute of Medicine (IOM) assess PEPFAR's performance and its effects on health.[2] Specifically, the task was to evaluate progress in meeting prevention, care, and treatment targets; the impact of PEPFAR-supported HIV prevention, treatment, and care programs; the effects of PEPFAR on health systems; PEPFAR's efforts to address gender-specific aspects of HIV/AIDS; and the impact of PEPFAR on child health and welfare.

To conduct a rigorous assessment that took into account PEPFAR's complexity and varied contexts, the IOM committee employed a mix of methods using financial data, program monitoring indicators and clinical data, extensive document review, and primary data collection carried out through more than 400 semi-structured interviews and site visits. A range of stakeholders were interviewed in 13 PEPFAR partner countries, at the U.S. headquarters of PEPFAR, and at other institutions and multilateral agencies.

The availability of the data needed to address all the health outcomes and impacts in the mandate was limited, and few data sources exist that are comparable and comprehensive across all PEPFAR partner countries. Therefore, the evaluation relied on sources from which robust information could be gathered on subsets of countries and select components within programmatic areas. Then, by assessing convergence and consistency among findings from different yet complementary data sources and methods, the committee analyzed and interpreted the available data to develop reasonable conclusions and recommendations about performance, impact, and progress across the whole of PEPFAR.

---

[2] Lantos-Hyde Act of 2008 at §101(c), 22 U.S.C. 7611(c). The complete Statement of Task can be found in Appendix A.

EVALUATION CONCLUSIONS AND RECOMMENDATIONS

PEPFAR has made remarkable progress in meeting its aims, reflecting the U.S. government's commitment and capability to respond to humanitarian crises through the use of health and development assistance and health diplomacy. PEPFAR's efforts have saved and improved the lives of millions of people by supporting HIV prevention, care, and treatment services; meeting the needs of children affected by the epidemic; building capacity; strengthening systems; engaging with partner country governments and other stakeholders; increasing knowledge about the epidemic in partner countries; and ensuring that attention be paid to vulnerable populations in the response to HIV.

While PEPFAR has achieved great things, its work is unfinished. The committee offers several recommendations to improve the U.S. government's support for the global response to HIV. They appear below in bold text, each followed by an indication of the chapter in the report in which it appears, and where additional considerations for its implementation are also described.[3,4]

The recommendations are presented in this summary in four main areas: scaling up HIV programs, strengthening systems for the HIV response in partner countries, transitioning to a sustainable response in partner countries, and transforming knowledge management to improve effectiveness.

Scaling Up HIV Programs

PEPFAR has provided a "proof of principle" that HIV services can be successfully delivered on a large scale in countries with a high burden of disease and limited available resources and infrastructure.

PEPFAR has increased the availability of and access to HIV testing, counseling, and diagnosis; as a result, many individuals have learned their HIV status. PEPFAR has also made it possible for an increasing number of adults and children living with HIV to receive clinical care and treatment, including antiretroviral therapy, through an expansion of the number and geographic distribution of clinical care and treatment sites, training and support for providers, procurement and delivery of drugs, improvements

[3] The recommendations with their implementation considerations are compiled in Appendix B.

[4] The report is structured in four parts. Part I presents background information and details the evaluation's scope and approach. Part II discusses PEPFAR's organization and investment. Part III assesses programmatic activities serving both general and key populations as well as health systems strengthening. For pragmatic reasons the different program areas are discussed in separate chapters (Prevention, Care and Treatment, Children and Adolescents, Gender, and Health Systems Strengthening). However, each chapter also recognizes the inherent relatedness of these program areas in a continuum of services. Part IV examines the future role of the U.S. government in the global response, with themes of sustainability and knowledge management.

in laboratory services, and support for the adoption and implementation of national policies and guidelines in partner countries.

Despite such remarkable and substantial progress, ongoing challenges across the continuum of clinical care and treatment services must be addressed to achieve positive health outcomes for people living with HIV and to ensure that care and treatment programs are contributing to a sustainable HIV response. One critical need is to improve linkages from HIV counseling and testing to care and treatment and also to prevention services aimed at reducing HIV transmission. Another essential need is to improve retention and adherence among patients in care and treatment.

In addition to clinical care and treatment services, PEPFAR has also supported nonclinical care and support services for adults and has provided unprecedented support for programs for orphans and vulnerable children infected with or affected by HIV. However, these services span a diffuse array of activities and often lack the strategic development in program portfolios necessary to maximize contributions to defined outcomes.

> **To contribute to sustainable care and treatment programs in partner countries, PEPFAR should build on its experience and support efforts to develop, implement, and scale up more effective and efficient facility- and community-based service delivery models for the continuum of adult and pediatric testing, care, and treatment. These efforts should aim to enhance equitable access, improve retention, increase clinical and laboratory monitoring, ensure quality, and implement cost efficiencies.** (Chapter 6)

> **To assess PEPFAR-supported HIV care and treatment programs and to evaluate new service delivery models, the Office of the U.S. Global AIDS Coordinator[5] should support an enhanced, nested program monitoring effort in which additional longitudinal data on core outcomes for HIV-positive adults and children enrolled in care and treatment are collected and centrally reported from a coordinated representative sample across multiple countries and implementing partners.** (Chapter 6)

This effort would serve as a nested evaluation within routine program monitoring systems to allow for long-term operational assessment of performance and outcomes for care and treatment across a representative

[5] It is the committee's intent that actions recommended to be taken by the Office of the U.S. Global AIDS Coordinator (OGAC) should be carried out through PEPFAR's interagency coordination mechanism, which involves not only the OGAC staff but also the leadership and technical staff of the U.S. government implementing agencies.

sample of PEPFAR-supported programs. The aim would be to focus on key areas for the assessment and improvement of programs as PEPFAR supports innovations in service delivery and transitions to new models of implementation. Data collected and reported for this sample should be harmonized with existing data collection whenever possible. Priorities for longitudinal assessment should include quality measures; core outcomes related to clinical care and treatment, including those in key challenge areas such as adherence and retention; and outcomes related to the reduction of HIV transmission through biomedical and behavioral prevention interventions for people living with HIV. Program measures, such as service costs, that can provide valuable information to identify efficiencies and promote sustainable management should also be included.

> **To improve the implementation and assessment of nonclinical care and support programs for adults and children, including programs for orphans and vulnerable children, the Office of the U.S. Global AIDS Coordinator should shift its guidance from specifying allowable activities to instead specifying a limited number of key outcomes. The guidance should permit country programs to select prioritized outcomes to inform the selection, design, and implementation of their activities. The guidance should also specify how to measure and monitor the key outcomes.** (Chapters 6 and 7)

To enable this shift to a more outcomes-oriented approach, partner countries will need support and assistance to prioritize outcomes and target services. For orphans and vulnerable children in particular, PEPFAR should improve the targeted coverage and quality of services by more explicitly and narrowly defining eligibility for PEPFAR-supported services at the country program level based on country-specific assessments of needs.

While services for people living with HIV are one foundation for the sustainable management of an HIV response, prevention is also paramount as part of a balanced attempt to change the trajectory of the HIV epidemic. PEPFAR's support for the scale-up of HIV prevention activities has been a valuable contribution to the HIV response in partner countries. PEPFAR has become more flexible over time in its approach to prevention, shifting from required budgetary allocations for specific intervention approaches to enabling the activities it supports to be tailored according to a country's epidemiological information and the available evidence for intervention effectiveness. As a result, PEPFAR's prevention programming has evolved from a limited number of behavioral and biomedical interventions initially to a greatly expanded portfolio of supported interventions based on existing and emergent evidence. A notable and measurable success in prevention has come in the area of the prevention of mother-to-child transmission, in which PEPFAR support has made a major contribution toward meeting the needs of partner countries.

Targeting the specific populations that are vulnerable to HIV infection and transmission, which differ by country, is critical for prevention. Notwithstanding some restrictive U.S. and partner country policy and legal environments, PEPFAR has made progress in this area through its support for data collection in specific populations and for prevention and harm reduction programming; these efforts have resulted in positive effects for populations at elevated risk, including men who have sex with men, people who engage in sex work, people who inject drugs, and other populations identified as vulnerable. Populations at elevated risk remain an important focus for prevention programming, and they also continue to struggle with barriers to accessing care and treatment services.

PEPFAR has stated its ongoing commitment to overarching goals for prevention. However, PEPFAR lacks clear objectives for outcomes across all types of prevention interventions. Achieving measurable intermediate outcomes for prevention efforts is important for PEPFAR to achieve its goals for reducing HIV transmission. However, there are limitations, not unique to PEPFAR, in the methods for appropriately measuring the outcomes of prevention interventions and in the available evidence for effectiveness for some types of intervention. These challenges are particularly salient for behavioral and structural interventions, especially for the prevention of sexual transmission, the primary global driver of HIV infection. An effective response requires responsiveness not only to the available evidence on intervention effectiveness, but also to the epidemiological evidence about the drivers of the epidemic. Given that behavioral and structural drivers will not be addressed through biomedical approaches alone, PEPFAR can contribute to a more effective HIV response by serving as a platform for innovation to help fill this gap in the availability of effective interventions and of appropriate approaches to assess prevention interventions. This would allow for a more balanced and comprehensive operational approach to developing, implementing, and evaluating prevention portfolios that are aligned with the drivers of epidemics and the needs for prevention services.

To contribute to the sustainable management of the HIV epidemic in partner countries, PEPFAR should support a stronger emphasis on prevention. The prevention response should prioritize the reduction of sexual transmission, which is the primary driver of most HIV infections, while maintaining support for interventions targeted at other modes of transmission. The response should incorporate an approach balanced among biomedical, behavioral, and structural interventions that is informed by epidemiological data and intervention effectiveness evidence. PEPFAR should sup-

port advances in prevention science to expand the availability of effective interventions where knowledge is lacking. (Chapter 5)

PEPFAR has articulated overarching aims for addressing gender-related factors that influence the HIV epidemic and response. In particular, PEPFAR has placed a strong emphasis on addressing gender-based violence, an important underlying driver of vulnerability in the HIV epidemic. PEPFAR's efforts have evolved from a focus on the HIV-related needs and vulnerabilities of women and girls to a more comprehensive focus that aims to also address the vulnerabilities of men and boys that arise as a result of social and cultural norms in partner countries about gender and sexuality. PEPFAR's gender efforts have scaled up slowly over time, in an ad hoc fashion, with little strategic guidance to facilitate comprehensive country portfolios that address gender norms and inequities and that incorporate gender-focused objectives within prevention, care, and treatment programs to improve service access, coverage, and quality for both men and women.

To achieve PEPFAR's stated aim of addressing gender norms and inequities as a way to reduce HIV risk and increase access to HIV services, the Office of the U.S. Global AIDS Coordinator (OGAC) should develop and clearly state objectives and desired outcomes for gender-focused efforts. OGAC should issue guidance for how to operationalize, implement, monitor, and evaluate activities and interventions to achieve these objectives. (Chapter 8)

Despite remarkable scale-up in PEPFAR partner countries, an all-encompassing challenge is the substantial remaining unmet need for all services and programs that are part of an effective response to HIV. For example, for antiretroviral therapy, fundamental challenges are posed by the large numbers of currently enrolled patients who need to be maintained, the patients who are currently eligible but not yet enrolled, and the potential for expansion of eligibility under new World Health Organization guidelines. For infants, children, and adolescents, service coverage in the continuum of testing, care, and treatment remains proportionally much lower than the coverage for adults. Programs for orphans and vulnerable children and adolescents also struggle to cover service needs in this population. Across HIV programs, an important goal for the future is for PEPFAR to work with partner countries and global partners, in the face of limited resources, to sustain the gains made and to continue to make progress in controlling the HIV epidemic.

Strengthening Health Systems for the HIV Response in Partner Countries

PEPFAR has made considerable contributions in many areas of health system functioning in partner countries. Its substantial support for laboratory strengthening has had fundamentally positive effects for the response to HIV and has been leveraged to improve the functioning of entire health systems. PEPFAR has also improved the functional components of systems that supply essential medications and other commodities critical for providing all health services. Despite this improvement, in many countries challenges remain with the consistency and reliability of supply chain functioning, which in turn affects sustainability and cost-effectiveness. PEPFAR has expanded the health workforce with the capacity to provide HIV services in partner countries; these contributions are now transitioning appropriately to more pre-service education and training, including initiatives for strengthening academic institutions, degree programs, and long-course trainings in countries. PEPFAR has also supported individual and organizational capacity building for leadership and for program and financial management across the governmental, private, and civil society sectors.

PEPFAR has supported the development and strengthening of national health information systems, with investments primarily in training and analytics, supply chain management, human resource information systems, laboratory management systems, patient record management systems, and electronic health records. When PEPFAR began, its focus on collecting data to monitor and report on the implementation of its programs led, when this capability was not available in partner countries, to PEPFAR-specific systems; these systems are now being increasingly aligned with national data collection for health as well as with global HIV indicators. Tensions remain between PEPFAR's data requirements for its own accountability and its aims to align with data collection for national systems, but PEPFAR is seeking to resolve this issue through enhanced support to strengthen national health information systems.

In service delivery, PEPFAR's impressive achievements represent the success of a largely disease-specific approach. In some countries, an early emphasis on increasing service volume to meet service delivery targets did not always facilitate service integration. Many stakeholders in partner countries have identified a need for greater integration of HIV services into the general health system. This is now an articulated goal for PEPFAR, but best practices for effective and efficient service integration are needed to facilitate scale-up. Another important need is ensuring the ongoing quality of services provided and programs implemented, especially through future transitions in implementation models for PEPFAR-supported programs.

PEPFAR's reauthorization created strategic opportunities for more formal support of health systems strengthening as a key contributor to sustainability in partner countries, encompassing all six building blocks in the World Health Organization framework: medical products and technologies, workforce, leadership and governance, financing, information systems, and service delivery.

> **To support the delivery of HIV-related services, make progress toward sustainable management of the HIV response, and contribute to other health needs, PEPFAR should continue to implement and leverage efforts that have had positive effects within partner country health systems. PEPFAR should maintain efforts in all six building blocks but have a concerted focus on areas that will be most critical for sustaining the HIV response, especially workforce, supply chain, and financing.** (Chapter 9)

Enhancing service delivery through existing local systems and long-term infrastructure development will continue to strengthen and expand the capacity of health and other systems to provide the services that are fundamental to an effective response to HIV, one that can meet the current and future trajectory of need. There is a need for future U.S. government investments to support long-term capacity building that fosters the placement and retention of trained personnel in partner countries to accelerate progress toward country ownership and sustainability.

> **To contribute to a country-owned and sustainable HIV response, the Office of the U.S. Global AIDS Coordinator should develop a comprehensive plan for long-term capacity building in partner countries. The plan should target four key areas: service delivery, financial management, program management, and knowledge management.** (Chapter 10)

Transitioning to a Sustainable Response in Partner Countries

PEPFAR has increasingly supported partner countries in the development of national frameworks, policies, and strategic plans. Participating in an intergovernmental planning process with partner country governments—one that includes multisectoral government participation as well as other local stakeholders and external donors—is one of the primary tools that PEPFAR uses to enhance leadership and governance and to support country ownership through mutual transparency, responsibility, and accountability. The U.S. government, like all donors, has its own considerations and requirements for funding decisions, but PEPFAR has made progress in making its considerations a part of joint planning processes rather than a displacement of country priorities. This joint planning includes both local processes for national plans as well as PEPFAR-specific processes, especially Partnership Frameworks. By necessity, PEPFAR will gradually cede control as partner countries adopt more dominant roles in setting strategic priorities for investments in their HIV response and in accounting for their results.

OGAC has recently articulated PEPFAR's understanding of country ownership and provided clarity about ways to mutually assess progress toward sustainability of a more country-led response. This transition to sustainability will be affected by many criteria and decisions, most of which will vary by country. Transitioning will take time; it cannot be achieved on a prescribed generic timeline across PEPFAR. Along the way, major dilemmas, such as differences in how to prioritize services and target populations, will require mutual resolution. In addition, transitioning to new models of PEPFAR support, including less direct support for service delivery and more technical assistance and systems strengthening, is part of a reasonable strategy for achieving sustainable management, but it also carries the inherent risks that in the transition period the same level of targets and access to services will not be achievable and that the quality of services, programs, and data may diminish. At the same time, greater embedding of HIV services in national health systems may offer opportunities for better integration of care, greater efficiencies, and broader health benefits.

There is strong leadership in partner countries for the HIV response, but many of these countries rely heavily—and in some cases almost exclusively—on U.S. bilateral assistance or the Global Fund. This reliance creates fragility and the possibility that the response would be disrupted if funding were discontinued or severely reduced. It is not realistic to expect that partner countries would be able to independently finance the entirety of HIV programming as it is currently implemented, and the critical importance of a global commitment to the HIV response remains. Yet, this does not abate the importance of partner country governments finding ways to reduce the fragility and dependence of their response by increasing their funding contributions, diversifying the sources of external funding that they receive, and making strategic, albeit difficult, decisions about the efficient use of available resources.

Building on the Partnership Framework implementation process, PEPFAR should continue to work with partner country governments and other stakeholders to plan for sustainable management of the response to HIV. PEPFAR should support and participate in comprehensive country-specific planning that includes the following:

- **Ascertain the trajectory of the epidemic and the need for prevention, care and treatment, and other services.**
- **Identify gaps, unmet needs, and fragilities in the current response.**
- **Estimate costs of the current response and project resource needs for different future response scenarios.**
- **Develop plans for resource mobilization to increase and diversify funding, including internal country-level funding sources.**
- **Encourage and participate in country-led, transparent stakeholder coordination and sharing of information related to funding, activities, and data collection and use.**
- **Establish and clearly articulate priorities, goals, and benchmarks for progress.** (Chapter 10)

PEPFAR is not alone in trying to achieve locally led, sustainable health and development objectives. Contributing stakeholders, including partner countries, will need to set priorities and allocate resources, based on mutually agreed-upon principles, to achieve a strategic and ethical balance between maintaining current coverage and expanding to address unmet needs. Ongoing support in partner countries to strengthen capacity for decision making informed by evidence will be needed to ensure that gains are not lost in achieving sustainable management of HIV programs, equitable access to services for those who are most in need, and sustainable control of the HIV epidemic.

Transforming Knowledge Management to Improve Effectiveness

PEPFAR's ability to generate, use, and disseminate knowledge is fundamental for program management and improvement and, ultimately, for the sustainability of PEPFAR's efforts. PEPFAR has made strong efforts in this area, often at levels not seen in other development initiatives, by creating a program monitoring data collection system to track activities and program results; supporting epidemiologic and surveillance activities; strengthening partner country health information systems; implementing various program evaluation approaches; and supporting some research across a wide range of technical areas. PEPFAR has generally utilized the resulting knowledge to drive program activities, implement evidence-informed interventions, and make modifications as new knowledge and scientific evidence have emerged. Yet, there are key areas where the information needed to assess efforts and guide future activities is not sufficient or is not available in a manner that facilitates use.

PEPFAR's indicators, like many program monitoring systems, are focused primarily on outputs, such as the number of individuals provided with a service. These serve an important function to monitor implementation of activities but do not reflect quality, efficiency, or effectiveness. Measuring program progress and effectiveness is not always best achieved through program monitoring systems. Therefore, strategic and coordinated evaluation and research are also critical activities that complement program monitoring indicators in order to assess meaningful outcomes and to continually improve the effectiveness and impact of PEPFAR investments. In addition, support for epidemiological data collection through surveillance and special studies in partner countries, which has been a cornerstone of PEPFAR's contribution, continues to be fundamental to supporting joint planning with partner countries.

PEPFAR would benefit from a more purposeful and strategic determination of which internal and external stakeholders need to know what information, at what level of the PEPFAR operational infrastructure, covering what scope of PEPFAR's efforts, and with what frequency. The limited personnel, time, and financial resources for knowledge management could then be allocated to monitoring, evaluation, research, and dissemination activities that meet these needs, while reducing the burden of collecting and reporting data and other information that is not useful.

PEPFAR will need to transform its approach to knowledge management in order to adapt to a transition from direct support for delivery of services and programs to increased support and technical assistance for systems strengthening, capacity building, and sustainable management of the response by partner country stakeholders. An investment now to develop reliable, credible approaches to assess the effectiveness of these efforts will be needed to document future progress and to continually improve future efforts. The ability to attribute results by counting services provided or beneficiaries reached will become less relevant; in fact, direct attribution will no longer be an appropriate expectation for accountability. PEPFAR could seize this opportunity to work with others in the global health and development assistance communities to develop appropriate ways to assess contributions to the improved performance and effectiveness of national efforts.

The Office of the U.S. Global AIDS Coordinator (OGAC) should develop a comprehensive knowledge management framework, including a program monitoring and evaluation strategy, a prioritized and targeted research portfolio, and systems for knowledge dissemination. This framework should adapt to emerging needs to

assess PEPFAR's models of implementation and contribution to sustainable management of the HIV response in partner countries. (Chapter 11)

This knowledge management framework will require that PEPFAR implement and strategically allocate resources for the following:

A. To better document PEPFAR's progress and effectiveness, OGAC should refine its program monitoring and evaluation strategy to streamline reporting and to strategically coordinate a complementary portfolio of evaluation activities to assess outcomes and effects that are not captured well by program monitoring indicators. Efforts should support innovation in methodologies and measures where needed. Both monitoring and evaluation should be specifically matched to clearly articulated data sources, methods, and uses at each level of PEPFAR's implementation and oversight.

OGAC's program monitoring reporting structure can be streamlined by focusing on program improvement at the partner level, monitoring at the country level, and strategic oversight of accountability for contribution at the headquarters level. To reduce duplicative efforts and investments in its evaluation portfolio, OGAC should coordinate among country programs to strategically plan and coordinate a subset of evaluations designed not only to be useful at the country level but also to enable comparability across programs and countries in order to assess performance and inform improvements across PEPFAR.

B. To contribute to filling critical knowledge gaps that impede effective and sustainable HIV programs, OGAC should continue to redefine permitted research within PEPFAR by developing a prioritized portfolio with articulated activities and methods. The planning and implementation process at the country and program level should inform and be informed by the research portfolio, which should focus on research that will improve the effectiveness, quality, and efficiency of PEPFAR-supported activities and will also contribute to the global knowledge base on implementation of HIV/AIDS programs.

PEPFAR's scope, scale, and experience mean that it is uniquely situated as a platform for research to spur innovation and to address knowledge gaps that can undermine the effective planning, implementation, and measurement of the effectiveness of programs at scale. Research and evaluation activities that emphasize in-country local participation and expertise can also enhance local capacity and contribute to country ownership.

C. To maximize the use of knowledge created within PEPFAR, OGAC should develop systems and processes for routine, active transfer and dissemination of knowledge both within and external to PEPFAR. As one component, OGAC should institute a data-sharing policy, developed through a consultative process. The policy should identify the data to be included and ensure that these stipulated data and results generated by PEPFAR or through PEPFAR-supported activities are made available in a timely manner to PEPFAR stakeholders, external evaluators, the research community, and other interested parties.

PEPFAR would benefit from building on its most successful current mechanisms for sharing data, information, and knowledge to develop more systematic documentation and dissemination; there is a particular need to more effectively facilitate the direct transfer of experiences, best practices, and lessons learned across countries, implementing partners, and sites.

CONCLUSION

PEPFAR is an unprecedented initiative implemented on behalf of the U.S. citizenry, with vast bilateral investment from the U.S. government. Its dynamism can be seen in its evolving scope and implementation, the changing context in which it operates, and its deepening interrelationship with health diplomacy. PEPFAR's support for HIV prevention, care, and treatment has had major positive effects on the health and well-being of individual beneficiaries, on institutions and systems in partner countries, and on the overall global response to HIV. In addition to the positive effects of PEPFAR's support for services, PEPFAR is generally recognized as providing good technical assistance; being a flexible donor that fills gaps and supports innovation within country structures; contributing to addressing the challenging nature of concentrated epidemics; advancing global expectations for performance measurement and accountability; and contributing to the global knowledge base. PEPFAR has also contributed to shaping global health policy and action for HIV and potentially other areas of health and development.

The committee's overall assessment is that PEPFAR has played a transformative role with its contribution to the global response to HIV. In the course of this evaluation, the committee heard repeatedly across countries the pride, gratitude, and appreciation expressed by partner country governments, implementing partners, providers working in PEPFAR-supported facilities and programs, and community-based and civil society organizations representing the beneficiaries of PEPFAR programs. PEPFAR was described as a lifeline, and people credit PEPFAR for restoring hope.

The future of PEPFAR's contribution lies in a new direction. PEPFAR is transitioning to new implementation models that enhance systems and capacity while facilitating capable leadership in partner countries to sustainably manage the response to HIV. This new era may not be one of rapid, dramatic results. Yet, if it is successful, then PEPFAR has the potential to again transform the way health assistance is envisioned and implemented, with ultimate long-term positive effects for health and well-being.

Main Messages

4

U.S. Funding for the PEPFAR Initiative

MAIN MESSAGES

- The U.S. Government (USG) is the largest donor to the global HIV epidemic, and PEPFAR's investment represents an historic contribution in countries with few resources and a great need for support in their response to HIV.
- The greater part of PEPFAR's funding has always gone to support programs and activities implemented in partner countries. Consistent with one aspect of PEPFAR's articulated strategy to move toward sustainability, more PEPFAR funding over time has been directed to local prime partners. Based on an analysis of a subset of data and countries, the increase in local prime partner funding has been driven primarily by increased funding to nongovernmental entities based in partner countries; the proportion of funding to partner country governments as prime partners has remained relatively stable over time.
- PEPFAR is increasingly emphasizing a range of efforts to more strategically and efficiently use its resources through the generation and use of economic and financial data; the allocation of resources based on anticipated impact; improved collaboration with partner country governments, other donors, and the Global Fund to align priorities and programs; and streamlining of business processes. PEPFAR has started to see some gains from these efforts. Continuing to identify and implement opportunities for more strategic and efficient use of resources will be critical for making progress toward optimal return on investment in the response to HIV in partner countries.
- Because of limitations in the available financial data, it was difficult to fully assess the amount and distribution by program area and partner type of the annual direct investment of PEPFAR in partner countries. PEPFAR would benefit from the collection and reporting of financial data that not only serves for accounting purposes, but also are more closely aligned with programmatic data and program implementation. These data are critical for PEPFAR and external stakeholders to more

easily and effectively understand how well PEPFAR is being implemented and how PEPFAR's investment relates to both the targets and goals of PEPFAR-supported programs and the broader goal of transitioning to more sustainable management of the response to HIV in partner countries.

5

Prevention

MAIN MESSAGES

Overall

- PEPFAR's support for the scale-up of HIV prevention activities across prevention modalities has been an achievement and a contribution to the response to the epidemic in partner countries. Within PEPFAR there has been an evolution in prevention programming, from an initial focus on a limited number of behavioral and biomedical interventions, to an expansion of prevention portfolios to reflect both existing and emergent evidence-based approaches.
- Although PEPFAR has articulated a commitment to overarching goals for prevention, PEPFAR lacks clear target outcomes and objectives across all prevention modalities; this is especially the case for behavioral and structural interventions for prevention of sexual transmission, the primary global driver of HIV infection. To achieve its overall goal of reducing new infections and stopping the spread of the epidemic, PEPFAR will need a more comprehensive and balanced approach, with greater clarity in its operational guidance and mechanisms to support the development, implementation, monitoring, and evaluation of prevention portfolios in country programs that are aligned with the drivers of epidemics and the needs for prevention services. Greater attention to developing appropriate approaches to assess the effectiveness of prevention interventions across all modalities and modes of transmission would contribute to this more balanced and comprehensive operational approach.
- There are limitations to measuring the effects of prevention programs across modalities, and in particular for behavioral and structural interventions. These limitations are not unique to PEPFAR and a substantial increase in attention and effort will be required to address them, yet more comprehensively identifying and understanding the outputs, coverage, and outcomes of prevention interventions would be of immense value in accurately assessing and documenting the impact of prevention efforts. Across modalities, measuring and achieving key intermediate outcomes for prevention efforts is as important a goal for PEPFAR as achieving estimated impact on the number of infections averted.

Prevention of Sexual Transmission

- Interventions targeted at prevention of sexual transmission, including biomedical, behavioral, and structural interventions, are all critical components of a balanced and comprehensive prevention portfolio. Yet, within PEPFAR, there is disproportionately less program monitoring data and rigorous research evidence available on these interventions, especially behavioral and structural interventions, than on prevention of mother-to-child transmission (PMTCT) and other biomedical prevention programs. As a result, the committee was unable to assess the effectiveness or determine the outcomes or impact across partner countries of PEPFAR's efforts to reduce sexually transmitted HIV infections. There is a critical need for improved application of advances in social and behavioral science–based research and evaluation science for prevention to determine the most effective combination of prevention interventions in diverse country contexts. Given the scale of its programs and its commitment to implementation research, PEPFAR can contribute to a more effective HIV response by serving as a platform for innovation to fill the gap in knowledge and availability of effective interventions.
- There is recognition in PEPFAR of the important role of efforts for sex workers as a part of the national response in both concentrated and generalized epidemics. There are some examples of success as a result of PEPFAR-supported activities for this population, and increased flexibility over time for prevention budgeting and programming has enabled country programs to more readily plan activities for sex workers.
- Over time PEPFAR has increasingly supported data collection efforts and prevention programming for men who have sex with men, which PEPFAR has recently codified in programmatic guidance. Men who have sex with men are recognized as an important population for prevention and other PEPFAR-supported programming.

Prevention of Mother-to-Child Transmission

- PEPFAR support for scale-up of services for PMTCT has made a major contribution to meet the need in partner countries. Integration of PMTCT into maternal and child health is occurring and is a sign of evolution of the program. However, integration at the facility level with other services is variable, and the link between PMTCT and antiretroviral therapy for both women and children is still a challenge.

Prevention with People Who Inject Drugs

- PEPFAR has been increasingly instrumental in facilitating and supporting some harm reduction approaches in countries with epidemics for which injection drug use is a major or emerging driver. Notwithstanding restrictive U.S. and partner country policy and legal environments, a positive effect of these activities and programs is being seen in countries in which PEPFAR works, but substantial unmet need remains for harm reduction and other services for this population.

Recommendation Presented in This Chapter

Recommendation 5-1 To contribute to the sustainable management of the HIV epidemic in partner countries, PEPFAR should support a stronger emphasis on prevention. The prevention response should prioritize the reduction of sexual transmission, which is the primary driver of most HIV infections, while maintaining support for interventions targeted at other modes of transmission. The response should incorporate an approach balanced among biomedical, behavioral, and structural interventions that is informed by epidemiological data and intervention effectiveness evidence. PEPFAR should support advances in prevention science to expand the availability of effective interventions where knowledge is lacking.

Further considerations for implementation of this recommendation:

- PEPFAR has made a commitment to overarching goals for prevention and for achieving an AIDS-free generation, but this does not constitute a long-term prevention strategy that clearly states prevention objectives and the pathways to achieving them. The following elements will be critical for a more comprehensive strategy to achieve successful execution of prevention programs:
  - PEPFAR should continue to enhance its efforts to involve partner country stakeholders and incorporate country-specific epidemiology, context, and priorities in planning appropriately matched prevention programs that achieve a balanced approach to HIV prevention across the available modalities. To provide greater technical and operational clarity, the Office of the U.S. Global AIDS Coordinator (OGAC) should provide mechanisms to support the development, implementation, and monitoring of comprehensive prevention portfolios, including how to determine what populations need which directed prevention activities in which settings. Areas of prevention where current interventions are successful and effective, such as PMTCT, should be continued and scaled up to ensure access, coverage, and quality. As new PEPFAR-supported prevention activities are adopted, OGAC should communicate its objectives and the methods for introducing or scaling up with specified populations.
  - OGAC should improve mechanisms to collect and incorporate evidence on the effectiveness of prevention activities implemented in partner countries. The key components for future assessment

and evaluation of HIV prevention should include need, coverage of need, quality of services provided, and behavioral and epidemiological outcomes. OGAC should provide clearly defined process and outcome measures as well as impact assessment methods to evaluate progress.

- PEPFAR's prevention strategy should include balanced support for innovation, research, and evaluation to contribute to the evolving evidence base and advance understanding of the effectiveness of interventions within all prevention modalities. To define and ensure this balance, OGAC should, through its existing mechanisms, convene and use expertise spanning behavioral, structural, and biomedical prevention intervention approaches. PEPFAR-supported research and evaluation activities should employ appropriate methodologies and study designs, without unduly emphasizing random assignment designs. PEPFAR should support innovations in prevention science methodologies where needed to achieve its programmatic research aims (see also Recommendation 11-1).

6

Care and Treatment

MAIN MESSAGES

HIV Counseling and Testing

- PEPFAR's efforts have led to a considerable achievement in increasing the availability of and access to HIV testing, counseling, and diagnosis. As a result, many more individuals have learned their HIV status and, if positive, been linked to clinical services. However, challenges remain in achieving adequate coverage of testing services, especially in scaling up and improving access to testing for infants and children and testing for pregnant women who do not attend antenatal care or deliver in health facilities. For those who test positive, challenges also remain in consistently ensuring they are linked to care and treatment as well as to prevention services to reduce HIV transmission. Overcoming these challenges and continuing to make progress in HIV counseling and testing will be a critical factor in achieving a successful comprehensive response to HIV.

HIV Care and Treatment Services

- PEPFAR has made a major contribution to increasing the number of people living with HIV who are in care and on antiretroviral therapy (ART) through the expansion of the number and geographic distribution of care and treatment sites, the training of providers, the procurement and delivery of drugs, improvements in laboratory services, and support for the adoption and implementation of national policies and guidelines in partner countries. Support for care and treatment programs is a success that has contributed to saving lives and improving the quality of life for people living with HIV in PEPFAR partner countries.
- Retention and adherence are critical and persistent challenges in PEPFAR-supported HIV care and treatment programs. Understanding the factors that contribute to the lack of retention and the most effective strategies to improve it is needed to fully maximize the role of care and treatment in a sustainable HIV/AIDS response.

- PEPFAR has made a tremendous contribution to a wide variety of clinical and nonclinical care and support services, beyond the provision of antiretroviral therapy, through scale-up of services and programs in facilities and communities and through support for partner country policies, guidelines, and protocols. However, in the area of nonclinical care and support in particular, services span a diffuse range of activities across countries and it is difficult to assess their effects. Information is lacking on the distribution of services, the intended outcomes, how well the services are matched to population and subpopulation needs, and the effectiveness of these services.
- The particular importance of efforts to address HIV and tuberculosis (TB) is well-recognized within PEPFAR and in partner countries, given that TB is a common co-infection and a leading cause of death for people living with HIV. PEPFAR has increasingly supported the integration and coordination of screening, diagnosis, and referrals or other linkages to treatment for both infections. PEPFAR has also made a notable contribution in its support for advancing policies and systems for TB/HIV integration in partner countries. However, progress in this area has come more slowly than in other clinical services for HIV, and challenges persist in achieving adequate coverage of both HIV screening for TB patients and TB screening for HIV patients, as well as in ensuring and monitoring subsequent referral and retention in treatment for both infections. Concerted efforts in this area will be critical for reducing mortality from TB/HIV as part of an effective response to HIV.
- The expansion of treatment has an ancillary effect of increasing drug resistance. The earlier that ART programs were implemented in a region, the more drug resistance is present. Because of the limited availability of second-line antiretroviral drugs in resource-limited settings, as drug resistance increases, the need for an expanded pharmaceutical arsenal for effective treatment intensifies. The emergence of HIV drug resistance is cause for greater efforts to improve the effectiveness and expand the implementation of adherence support, treatment failure and drug resistance monitoring strategies, and treatment options in resource-limited settings.
- The ability to assess the impact of PEPFAR-supported care and treatment programs across countries and partners is restricted by limitations in the available data. The available program-wide output measures provide a sense of the growth of PEPFAR-supported treatment programs over time but do not provide an understanding of the distribution of those services in populations of interest and do not provide measures of effectiveness and outcomes. It was a missed opportunity not to invest more resources earlier in standardized, realistic, and useful monitoring of outcomes.

Ongoing Challenge of Coverage

- Despite progress in the availability of and access to HIV services, there remains a large unmet need for care and treatment in PEPFAR partner countries. Intrinsic limitations of the health system infrastructure and other systems involved in the response continue to pose barriers to the delivery of care and treatment services, including nonclinical care, clinical care, clinical and laboratory monitoring, and antiretroviral therapy.
- Treatment of infants and children remains a persistent challenge across the continuum of care. The main barriers, especially for infants, come at the stages of testing and diagnosis, linkages to care and treatment, and timely initiation of therapy. Limitations in health systems for support of pediatric HIV services are also a major factor. PEPFAR has contributed to increasing pediatric treatment, but the coverage of pediatric HIV remains proportionally much lower than the coverage for adults, despite the goal in the reauthorization legislation to provide care and treatment services in partner countries to children in proportion to their percentage within the HIV-infected population.

Sustainability of HIV Treatment

- A fundamental challenge for the sustainability of care and treatment across PEPFAR partner countries is how to maintain those currently enrolled in care and treatment, address the care and treatment needs for the many currently eligible patients who are not yet enrolled, and plan for those who will become eligible in the future, especially as changing World Health Organization (WHO) guidelines are adopted and implemented. There is a critical need for PEPFAR to work with partner countries and other global partners to sustain the gains made, to continue to make progress in achieving greater coverage, and to ensure the ongoing quality of services provided and programs implemented. Given the realities of resource constraints and the possible flattening or decreasing of external resources, contributing stakeholders will need to allocate resources with a strategic and ethical balance among coverage priorities.

Recommendations Presented in This Chapter

Recommendation 6-1: To improve the implementation and assessment of nonclinical care and support programs for adults and children, including programs for orphans and vulnerable children,[1] the Office of the U.S. Global AIDS Coordinator should shift its guidance from specifying allowable activities to instead specifying a limited number of key outcomes. The guidance should permit country programs to select priori-

[1] The discussion of programs for orphans and vulnerable children leading to this aspect of this recommendation can be found in Chapter 7.

tized outcomes to inform the selection, design, and implementation of their activities. The guidance should also specify how to measure and monitor the key outcomes.

Further considerations for implementing this recommendation:

- Outcomes for consideration should reflect the aims of care and support programs, which are to optimize quality of life, promote health, slow the progression of AIDS, and reduce HIV-related complications and mortality. Other outcomes of importance for the performance and effectiveness of care and support programs include measures of quality of services and equitable access to services.
- PEPFAR U.S. mission teams should work with partner country stakeholders and implementers to assess country-specific needs and to select a subset of the core key outcomes to focus on when planning, selecting, and developing evidence-informed activities and programs for implementation.
- The Office of the U.S. Global AIDS Coordinator (OGAC) should provide general guidance for country programs on continuous program evaluation and quality improvement to help them measure and monitor achievement of the key outcomes. This guidance may include, for example, template evaluation plans and methodological guidance. To allow for comparability across countries and programs, evaluation plans should include (but not be limited to) the defined indicators or other measures of the core key outcomes. Evaluations should emphasize the use of in-country local expertise (e.g., local implementing partners and subpartners and local academic institutions) to enhance capacity building and contribute to country ownership. (See also recommendations for PEPFAR's knowledge management in Chapter 11.)
- PEPFAR should develop a system for active dissemination and sharing of evaluation outcomes and best practices both within and across countries that is driven as much by country-identified needs for information as by opportunities for exchange of information identified by headquarters-level leadership and technical working groups. (See also recommendations for PEPFAR's knowledge management in Chapter 11.)

Recommendation 6-2: To contribute to sustainable care and treatment programs in partner countries, PEPFAR should build on its experience and support efforts to develop, implement, and scale up more effective and efficient facility- and community-based service delivery models for the continuum of adult and pediatric testing, care, and treatment. These efforts should aim to enhance equitable access, improve retention, increase clinical and laboratory monitoring, ensure quality, and implement cost efficiencies.

Further considerations for implementation of this recommendation:

- This recommendation should be implemented in coordination with recommendations and considerations discussed in Chapter 9 on health systems strengthening.
- PEPFAR should develop a system for active dissemination and sharing of best practices in service delivery both within and across countries. (See also recommendations for PEPFAR's knowledge management in Chapter 11.)

Recommendation 6-3: To assess PEPFAR-supported HIV care and treatment programs and to evaluate new service delivery models, the Office of the U.S. Global AIDS Coordinator should support an enhanced, nested program monitoring effort in which additional longitudinal data on core outcomes for HIV-positive adults and children enrolled in care and treatment are collected and centrally reported from a coordinated representative sample across multiple countries and implementing partners.

Further considerations for implementation of this recommendation:

- This activity would serve as a targeted, nested evaluation within routine program monitoring systems to allow for long-term operational assessment of performance and outcomes for care and treatment across a representative sample of PEPFAR-supported programs. The aim would be to focus on key areas for evaluation and improvement of programs going forward, including as PEPFAR supports innovations in service delivery and as PEPFAR-supported programs transition to new models of implementation.
- Data collected and reported for this sample should be harmonized with existing data collection whenever possible, including data already collected by implementing partners but not centrally reported (e.g., see the discussion of Tier 3 data in the implementation considerations for Recommendation 11-1A). Collaborative opportunities may be feasible with existing or new large-scale national and multi-country samples.
- This data-collection effort should be designed by first identifying and prioritizing the key questions that require longitudinal data and then focusing on relevant key outcomes with measures that are standardized across the sample. Priorities should include core outcomes related to clinical care and treatment, including adherence and retention; outcomes related to the reduction of HIV transmission through biomedical and behavioral prevention interventions for people living with HIV; quality measures; and program measures, such as the costs of services, that can help inform strategies for efficiencies, sustainable management, and resource planning for the trajectory of need.

- There may also be opportunities for an established data collection effort of this kind to serve as a synergistic platform for targeted implementation research studies in subset samples to assess innovations and advance those best practices that are most ready for translation and scale-up.
- In addition to implementing this approach prospectively, OGAC should explore working with and coordinating Track 1.0 partners to pool data for retrospective outcome analyses.

7

Children and Adolescents

MAIN MESSAGES

- PEPFAR has positively affected the lives of children and adolescents living with or affected by HIV. PEPFAR has contributed to major scale-up of services (orphans and vulnerable children [OVC], pediatric care and support, pediatric treatment, and prevention of mother-to-child transmission [PMTCT]) across delivery settings (facility-based, home-based, community-based, and family support). With its explicit focus on orphans and vulnerable children, PEPFAR has elevated attention to and investment in meeting the needs of this population through programs and services that are informed by evidence. PEPFAR has also been instrumental in facilitating partner country consideration and adoption of policies, laws, and guidelines on behalf of children and adolescents, including OVC policies and frameworks, policies for pediatric testing and treatment, and efforts to strengthen legislation and enforcement for child protection.
- Despite progress, there remain insufficiently met needs relating to the health and well-being of children and adolescents. Although it is not realistic to expect PEPFAR to meet all the need of children and adolescents in partner countries, there are particular areas where PEPFAR could strive to address these needs more fully. In particular, there remain gaps in coverage for PMTCT relative to PEPFAR's 85 percent goal; the coverage of pediatric HIV care and treatment remains proportionally much lower than the coverage for adults, despite the goal in the reauthorization legislation to provide care and treatment services in partner countries to children in proportion to their percentage within the HIV-positive population; and OVC programs struggle to adequately meet the needs of children, and adolescents in particular. Across program areas, there is also a need to plan for long-term sustainability of services and to build the capability of partner countries to continue the successes they have realized in addressing the needs of children and adolescents living with or affected by HIV.
- The ability to assess the impact of PEPFAR-supported programs for children and adolescents is restricted by limitations in the available data. There are data insufficiencies in three key areas directly related to PEPFAR programs: disaggregation both by sex and by age subgroups (e.g., less than 1 year, 1 to 5 years, and 6 to 17 years) to better understand what populations are receiving what services; baseline

and longitudinal data to follow children and families and the effects of the services they receive over time; and data on effectiveness and outcomes to help identify the most effective PEPFAR OVC programs and models. In addition, there is a lack of data about the total population of children "in need," in part because of a lack of clarity and consistency both across countries and across programs within countries in how the population eligible for PEPFAR-supported services is defined (i.e., which children are defined as "vulnerable" or "affected by HIV").

Recommendation Presented in This Chapter

Recommendation 7-1: To improve the implementation and assessment of nonclinical care and support programs for adults[1] and children, including programs for orphans and vulnerable children, the Office of the U.S. Global AIDS Coordinator should shift its guidance from specifying allowable activities to instead specifying a limited number of key outcomes. The guidance should permit country programs to select prioritized outcomes to inform the selection, design, and implementation of their activities. The guidance should also specify how to measure and monitor the key outcomes.

Further considerations for implementing this recommendation:

- For orphans and vulnerable children, the new OVC guidance and the ongoing developments for program evaluation already represent advances in addressing some of the challenges identified in this evaluation; this recommendation and the further considerations are intended to reinforce and further inform and support progress in achieving PEPFAR's goals for children and adolescents.
- Outcomes for consideration should be linked to the aims of OVC programs and therefore could include, for example, increased rates of staying in school, decreased excessive labor, reduced rates of exposure to further traumas, increased immunization completion, and increased coverage of HIV testing and treatment. With a continued focus on supporting developmentally informed programs, consideration should be given to identifying appropriate core outcomes for different age groups and for achieving developmental milestones. The program evaluation indicators currently being developed already offer a reasonable opportunity to link measures to core target outcomes for OVC programs.
- The core key outcomes should also include quality of services and measures to reflect the potential sustainability of programs.
- A shift to a more outcomes-oriented implementation model will re-

[1] The discussion of nonclinical care and support for adults leading to this aspect of this recommendation can be found in Chapter 6.

quire that partner countries receive support to define their prioritized outcomes and their target population and then to conduct baseline assessments so that progress toward outcomes can be measured.

- PEPFAR U.S. mission teams should work with partner country stakeholders and implementers to assess country-specific needs and to select a subset of the core key outcomes to focus on when planning, selecting, and developing evidence-informed activities and programs for implementation.
- Prioritization is critical in the presence of great need and finite resources. When planning with partner countries, PEPFAR should improve targeted coverage and the quality of supported services for affected children and adolescents not only by prioritizing outcomes and activities but also by more explicitly, clearly, and narrowly defining the eligibility for PEPFAR-supported services. This prioritization should be based on an assessment of country-specific needs with a process that consistently applies considerations and criteria across countries and programs. This prioritization should be done in coordination across program areas that address the needs and vulnerabilities of children and adolescents. These areas, which may target and serve a broader eligible population of children and adolescents than is determined for specific OVC programs, include care and treatment, PMTCT, other prevention services, and gender programs.
- To improve the targeted coverage and sustainability for children and adolescents, PEPFAR and its implementing partners should continue to enhance services through existing systems and infrastructure and to support national governments in expanding social support services and the workforce to meet the health, education, and psychosocial needs of affected children and adolescents.
- The Office of the U.S. Global AIDS Coordinator (OGAC) should provide general guidance for country programs on continuous program evaluation and quality improvement in order to measure and monitor the achievement of key outcomes. This may include, for example, template evaluation plans and methodological guidance. To allow for comparability across countries and programs, evaluation plans should include (but not be limited to) the defined indicators or other measures of the core key outcomes. Evaluations should emphasize the use of in-country local expertise (e.g., local implementing partners and sub-partners as well as local academic institutions) to enhance capacity building and contribute to country ownership. (See also recommendations for PEPFAR's knowledge management in Chapter 11.)
- PEPFAR should develop a system for the active dissemination and sharing of evaluation outcomes and best practices both within and across countries that is driven as much by country-identified needs for information as by opportunities for exchange of information identified by headquarters-level leadership and technical working groups. (See also recommendations for PEPFAR's knowledge management in Chapter 11.)

8

Gender

MAIN MESSAGES

- The scope and framing of PEPFAR's gender-focused efforts have evolved from a focus primarily on the HIV-related needs and vulnerabilities of women and girls to an expanded focus that aims to also address the vulnerabilities of men and boys (including men who have sex with men) that arise as a result of social and cultural norms about gender and sexuality. PEPFAR's efforts have also been scaled up over time from initial pilot programs to more central initiatives and country programming, with more financial and human resources devoted to them. This evolution is occurring in the context of a range of societal, cultural, economic, and other factors that affect gender norms in the countries in which PEPFAR is operating.
- The available data on differences between enrollment of women and men in antiretroviral therapy across countries indicate that there has been a successful scale-up of HIV treatment services for women as well as for men. Along with this success, both men and women continue to encounter barriers to accessing services. Men tend to have poorer health outcomes, in part due to enrollment in ART with later-stage illness.
- PEPFAR has placed a strong emphasis on addressing gender-based violence prevention and services. Continuing this focus is critical to changing one of the most important underlying structural drivers of vulnerability in the HIV epidemic.
- Over time, PEPFAR has increasingly supported policy, data collection, and programming efforts for men who have sex with men that vary by country context and local need and are informed by available evidence. PEPFAR has only recently codified this support in programmatic guidance. Men who have sex with men continue to struggle with barriers to accessing care and treatment services and remain an important population at elevated risk for prevention programming. In addition, a more holistic and integrated approach to activities for men who have sex with men could be used in future programming given that their needs and challenges cut across the continuum of HIV-related services.

- There are currently insufficient mechanisms and data to give either the Office of the U.S. Global AIDS Coordinator (OGAC) or country programs an adequate assessment of the effectiveness of gender-focused programming and its impact on societal norms and health disparities. There is a need for PEPFAR to develop an adequate approach, through both the program monitoring system and a coordinated effort of periodic evaluation and other activities, to adequately assess what efforts are being implemented and the outcomes of these efforts across the full range of its programmatic portfolio for gender-focused activities.

Overall Conclusion

- As PEPFAR's gender efforts have evolved and expanded, there have been positive effects of these efforts. However, the approach for how PEPFAR engages with gender-related factors that influence the HIV epidemic and response has been ad hoc. Although PEPFAR has articulated its framing of gender vulnerabilities and inequities and its overarching aims in its Gender and HIV Factsheet, it has not articulated the objectives that would need to be met in order to achieve those aims or the outcomes that would reflect success in these efforts. In addition, it does not provide guidance on intervention effectiveness or on approaches to establishing priorities for gender-focused efforts in different country settings and to developing strategic country-specific portfolios. Activities supported by PEPFAR central initiatives and through country operational planning vary widely in type and intensity of focus across the articulated gender aims and the populations that are addressed.

Recommendation Presented in This Chapter

Recommendation 8-1: To achieve PEPFAR's stated aim of addressing gender norms and inequities as a way to reduce HIV risk and increase access to HIV services, the Office of the U.S. Global AIDS Coordinator (OGAC) should develop and clearly state objectives and desired outcomes for gender-focused efforts. OGAC should issue guidance for how to operationalize, implement, monitor, and evaluate activities and interventions to achieve these objectives.

Further considerations for implementation of this recommendation:

- The objectives and guidance should be informed by the available evidence on how gender dynamics influence both HIV outcomes and the implementation of activities and services as well as by evidence on intervention effectiveness from the existing knowledge base, expert consultation, and experiences from pilot programs in partner countries.

- OGAC's guidance on gender-focused efforts should encompass programs specific to addressing gender norms and inequities and efforts to incorporate gender-focused objectives within prevention, care, and treatment activities.
- The development of guidance for gender-focused efforts should take advantage of lessons learned from the processes used for PEPFAR's recent updates to its guidance for prevention and orphans and vulnerable children (OVC) programs.
- PEPFAR U.S. mission teams should work with partner country stakeholders and implementers to strategically plan, select, develop, implement, and measure evidence-informed activities and programs to achieve the gender-focused objectives.
- Strategic implementation of gender-focused efforts will require strong technical leadership, and as such additional capacity in gender expertise will be needed at both the OGAC and U.S. mission team levels. If gender efforts are to be appropriately integrated into all the aspects of service delivery and effectively implemented, this capacity cannot be limited to gender-specific experts but should also be incorporated as part of the core competencies of mission team staff across PEPFAR's programmatic areas.
- As an engaged participant with other global and partner country stakeholders, through its implementation PEPFAR should contribute to generating evidence to inform gender-focused efforts through research and evaluation. (See also recommendations for PEPFAR's knowledge management in Chapter 11.)

- PEPFAR has supported training for management and leadership to build capacity for improved functioning of health systems with a variety of activities, including curriculum development, mentorship, and shorter-term trainings and workshops. However, the focus and outputs of these training efforts are varied, and it was difficult for the committee to determine the impact of these efforts from the data currently available.
- PEPFAR's capacity building approach has been holistic and includes developing human resources; strengthening financial management; and building organizational capacity at national, provincial, and district levels and across government, private, and civil society sectors. Despite these efforts, leadership and financial management capacity were frequently mentioned as challenges to effective HIV/AIDS responses.

Financing

- Data on partner country government expenditures for HIV/AIDS responses from National Health Accounts and National AIDS Spending Assessments for the 31 countries that are the focus of this evaluation were unavailable for many countries and years, making it difficult to examine trends in HIV/AIDS funding.
- Although there are nascent efforts in PEPFAR for the costing of services and the projecting of needs to help countries develop a costed HIV/AIDS response, PEPFAR has not yet systematically implemented assistance for partner countries to develop resource mobilization plans, conduct costing activities and resource projections, or identify funding needs.

Information Systems

- Despite initial PEPFAR-specific systems for program monitoring data, PEPFAR has worked with partner country governments to integrate and strengthen health information systems, including work that has strengthened partner country Laboratory Information Management Systems. However, ongoing support to strengthen partner country health information systems—and better alignment and integration with those systems—is needed to enhance timely data availability and quality for use in strategic program planning, resource allocation, and commodities procurement.

Medical Products and Technologies

- PEPFAR has improved the capacity of partner country governments to quantify, forecast, procure, store and warehouse, distribute, and track commodities, but challenges to assuring consistent and reliable supply chain functioning remain in many countries. These challenges are a common issue across countries and are not PEPFAR specific. Reliable supply chains will be critical for sustainable and cost-efficient HIV/AIDS responses and for avoiding disruptions to the clinical care and treatment of people living with HIV/AIDS.

- PEPFAR's laboratory efforts have had a fundamental and substantial impact on laboratory capacity in countries. This laboratory infrastructure and capacity has been, and can continue to be, leveraged to improve the functioning of countries' entire health systems.

Workforce

- PEPFAR's contribution to health workforces in partner countries has over time been appropriately directed to more pre-service production. Nonetheless, partner countries continue to have considerable need for health workforce development and retention. PEPFAR can contribute to fulfilling that need by leveraging and maximizing its investments in collaborative efforts to build the capacity of health professional training schools, which would improve the ability of countries to address not only HIV but also the dual burden of infectious and non-communicable diseases that many high-burden countries increasingly face. Adherence by partner countries to the Global Code of Practice on the International Recruitment of Health Personnel and followthrough on commitments to the Abuja Declaration could support both sustainability of their own health workforces and country ownership.

Service Delivery

- PEPFAR's impressive achievements in service delivery represent the success of a largely disease-specific approach, which had both positive and negative effects on partner country national health systems. In some countries, an early emphasis in PEPFAR implementation on increasing the volume of services to meet targets for service delivery resulted in disease-specific programming, which did not always facilitate service integration. PEPFAR has articulated the goal of increased integration of services and has had some success. Many stakeholders in partner countries have identified an interest or need for greater integration of HIV services into the general health system. The best practices for integrating services—such as those for HIV and tuberculosis, reproductive health, and primary care—need to be identified, evaluated, and scaled up.

Recommendation Presented in This Chapter

Recommendation 9-1: To support the delivery of HIV-related services, make progress toward sustainable management of the HIV response,

and contribute to other health needs, PEPFAR should continue to implement and leverage efforts that have had positive effects within partner country health systems. PEPFAR should maintain efforts in all six building blocks but have a concerted focus on areas that will be most critical for sustaining the HIV response, especially workforce, supply chain, and financing.

<u>Further considerations for implementation of this recommendation:</u>

- An important focus for PEPFAR's future activities and policies should be support for partner country capacity to locally produce and retain clinical, nonclinical, and management professionals whose training and scope of practice are appropriate and optimized for the tasks needed. The Medical Education and Nursing/Midwifery Education Partnership Initiatives have provided a starting point for the training of physicians and nurses; however, the training of associate clinician providers and other cadres will also be critical to the sustainable management of the response. In addition, PEPFAR needs to augment its efforts to build partner country capacity to track the placement of trained workers, to promote retention, and to develop long-term human resources plans. (See also the discussion and recommendation for capacity building in Chapter 10 on progress toward a sustainable response.)
- Building on the progress made through the public–private partnership with the Supply Chain Management System, PEPFAR should enhance and expand efforts with a greater focus on capacity building for accountable supply chain management in partner countries. The aim of this improved capacity should be to gradually shift to local or regional leadership, coordination, and management to ensure a reliable supply chain for essential medicines and commodities.
- Financing and leadership and governance are particularly critical for the sustainable management of the HIV response; this area is addressed in Recommendation 10-1 (see Chapter 10).
- To contribute to the knowledge base for health systems strengthening, PEPFAR should include this area in its research and evaluation agenda and its knowledge dissemination efforts. (See also recommendations for PEPFAR's knowledge management in Chapter 11.)

10

Progress Toward Transitioning to a Sustainable Response in Partner Countries

MAIN MESSAGES

- PEPFAR is actively engaging in activities and processes to transition to a more sustainable response in partner countries.
- Country ownership has not always had an agreed-upon definition once it was adopted from the development assistance lexicon and applied to PEPFAR. Recent efforts by the Office of the U.S. Global AIDS Coordinator (OGAC) have provided clarity for its definition and how partner countries should assess their achievement of its critical components.
- OGAC sees country ownership as a fundamental element of progress toward more sustainable management of the HIV/AIDS response by partner country governments and other relevant and engaged stakeholders in the country. In the transition to increasing country ownership, by necessity, PEPFAR will gradually cede control as partner countries adopt more dominant roles in setting strategic priorities for investments in their HIV response and in accounting for their results.
- The transition to a more country-led and -sustained response will take time; it cannot be achieved on a prescribed generic timeline for all PEPFAR countries. It will be affected by many criteria and decisions, which will vary by country, including where the country falls when it is evaluated across all four domains of political ownership and stewardship, institutional and community ownership, capabilities, and mutual accountability including finance in the OGAC-generated country ownership spectrum. Along the way, major dilemmas, such as differences in how to prioritize services and target populations will require mutual resolution. Inherent risks during the transition period may be reaching smaller targets, reduced service access, or the diminishing of the quality of services, programs, and data. At the same time, greater embedding of HIV services in national health systems may offer opportunities for better integration of care, greater efficiencies, and broader health benefits.

- PEPFAR has focused efforts on capacity building for all levels of stakeholders and attempts to bring many stakeholders to participate in the planning and oversight processes for Partnership Framework Implementation Plans for country-led response and leadership but with multisectoral participation. It will be a serious impediment to country ownership if the stakeholders expected to be involved in a country's HIV response do not all build their capacity.
- The over-reliance on external donor funding in partner countries creates funding fragility and the possibility that the HIV response would be critically disrupted if funding were to be discontinued or severely reduced. It is not realistic to expect that partner countries would be able to independently finance the entirety of HIV programming as it is currently implemented. Yet, this does not abate the importance of partner country governments finding ways to reduce the fragility and dependence of their response by increasing their funding contributions, diversifying the sources of external funding that they receive, and making efficient, albeit difficult, strategic decisions about the use of available resources. Even when countries are not able to substantially increase their own funding for HIV/AIDS or health, it is critically important that they demonstrate the leadership to understand their current and future needs by developing their own resources plan, including the responsibility they will undertake to mobilize the needed resources.

Recommendations Discussed in This Chapter

Recommendation 10-1: To contribute to a country-owned and sustainable HIV response, the Office of the U.S. Global AIDS Coordinator should develop a comprehensive plan for long-term capacity building in partner countries. The plan should target four key areas: service delivery, financial management, program management, and knowledge management.

<u>Further considerations for implementation of this recommendation:</u>

- In all four key areas, OGAC should invest more resources in initiatives for long-term capacity building and infrastructure development such as strengthening in-country academic institutions, degree programs, and long-course trainings, to improve in-country capacity and to accelerate progress toward country ownership and sustainability. These investments should foster the placement and retention of trained personnel in partner countries.
- These initiatives should be monitored routinely at the country level to assess progress and identify necessary modifications. Special periodic multi-country studies could be used to evaluate the outcome and impact of the PEPFAR capacity building initiative. To achieve this, OGAC should, using input from country programs, identify milestones toward achieving specified goals, define core metrics to assess capac-

ity building efforts, encourage innovative approaches through pilot initiatives, and develop tools to help country programs monitor and evaluate these efforts.

Recommendation 10-2: Building on the Partnership Framework implementation process, PEPFAR should continue to work with partner country governments and other stakeholders to plan for sustainable management of the response to HIV. PEPFAR should support and participate in comprehensive country-specific planning that includes the following:

- **Ascertain the trajectory of the epidemic and the need for prevention, care and treatment, and other services.**
- **Identify gaps, unmet needs, and fragilities in the current response.**
- **Estimate costs of the current response and project resource needs for different future response scenarios.**
- **Develop plans for resource mobilization to increase and diversify funding, including internal country-level funding sources.**
- **Encourage and participate in country-led, transparent stakeholder coordination and sharing of information related to funding, activities, and data collection and use.**
- **Establish and clearly articulate priorities, goals, and benchmarks for progress.**

Further considerations for implementing this recommendation:

- PEPFAR is not alone in trying to achieve locally-led, sustainable health and development objectives. Contributing stakeholders, including partner countries, will need mutually-agreed, principle-based resource allocation to achieve a strategic and ethical balance among the priorities of maintaining current coverage, expanding to meet existing unmet needs, and increasing coverage eligibility. Having processes in place to support this arduous decision making is a critical part of achieving sustainable HIV programs and sustainable management of the HIV epidemic in partner countries.
- Partners in developing resource mobilization plans and potential sources for more diverse funding and other resources could include national and subnational governments other bilateral donors, multilateral agencies, global and regional development banks, and private sector consultants.
- There may be learning opportunities at both headquarters and country level for PEPFAR and other U.S. government entities involved in development assistance to exchange strategies, best practices, and lessons learned for sustaining development objectives.

11

PEPFAR's Knowledge Management

MAIN MESSAGES

Informing Priorities for PEPFAR-Supported Programs

- Despite some exceptions, PEPFAR has implemented evidence-informed programs that have been modified as new knowledge and scientific evidence emerged. Target setting has been used to focus PEPFAR activities, program planning, and accountability. PEPFAR has utilized epidemiological and intervention effectiveness data to drive program activities.
- PEPFAR has provided financial and technical support for collecting epidemiological information in partner countries. This was widely seen as a positive contribution to inform decisions and priorities in planning the HIV/AIDS response and implementing HIV programs, encouraging and facilitating responsiveness to the epidemic and the needs in partner countries.

Program Monitoring Data

- PEPFAR's program monitoring indicator system has faced technological challenges limiting the ability of both PEPFAR and external stakeholders to utilize and access both current and historical trend data; resolving these challenges is critical for successful program monitoring.
- PEPFAR's program monitoring has evolved over time: the number of centrally reported indicators was reduced, indicators to monitor new program activities were introduced, and indicators identified as problematic, removed. PEPFAR needs a program monitoring strategy that can adapt over time to respond to feedback, reflect emerging program priorities, and accurately capture program activities and outcomes. However, this needs to be balanced with the reality that changes in indicators place a burden on partner country programs and limit comparability of data, hampering the ability to monitor trends.
- PEPFAR's current indicators do not capture sufficient information on its stated prioritized goals and activities and are focused primarily on

input and outputs. As a result, the program monitoring system has limited utility for determining the effectiveness of PEPFAR's efforts.

- The need to quickly measure results at the onset of PEPFAR contributed to the development of PEPFAR-specific data collection systems, which has limited harmonization with partner countries and the global HIV/AIDS community. More recently, the Office of the U.S. Global AIDS Coordinator (OGAC) has worked with other global actors to harmonize indicators and validate reporting. OGAC has modified the PEPFAR monitoring system to reduce reporting burden and improve alignment with partner country programs; however, further modifications could be made by eliminating PEPFAR-specific language in the indicator guidance; further reducing the reporting burden; improving indicator harmonization with global indicators; and advancing alignment with partner country data collection at the program level.
- There are some good examples of PEPFAR data use at the implementing partner, mission team, and headquarters (HQ) levels, but the preponderance of data collected does not seem to be routinely utilized. PEPFAR's requirement for collection and reporting of a large amount of program monitoring data places a large burden on implementing partners and mission teams that has limited the ability to analyze and use data.
- PEPFAR has invested in building the capacity of partner countries to plan for, collect, manage, and use HIV data, which has implications for the larger health system. As a result, PEPFAR has contributed to fostering a culture of evidence among partner countries.

PEPFAR-Supported Evaluation and Research

- The manner in which PEPFAR initially approached research activities was a missed opportunity to establish, from its inception, mechanisms to evaluate programs, assess impact, contribute to the global knowledge base, and develop in-country research capacity.
- PEPFAR has made progress in carrying out evaluation and research activities over time: moving from an early proscription against research, to using Targeted Evaluations and Public Health Evaluations to work within research restrictions, to the recent creation of what holds promise as a more useful process for establishing priorities, managing activities, documenting "what works," expanding PEPFAR's technical leadership, disseminating findings, and continually improving the effectiveness and impact of PEPFAR. Defining appropriate and allowable research activities within PEPFAR, however, was and remains a challenge, specifically clarity around the activities and aims for evaluation and research within PEPFAR.

Knowledge Transfer and Learning Within PEPFAR

- PEPFAR has successfully established and used a variety of mechanisms to transfer knowledge throughout PEPFAR; however, more progress is needed to address limitations in current systems and to establish formal mechanisms to systematically transfer experiences across countries, implementing partners, and sites. Without this, there will be missed opportunities to capitalize on best practices and internal lessons learned.

Knowledge Dissemination External to PEPFAR

- OGAC would benefit from developing a formal system to track and manage PEPFAR-funded dissemination products (e.g., publications, reports, abstracts, guidelines, and tools) from which to measure contribution to the global knowledge base, and the global HIV/AIDS community would benefit from a publicly available central repository of these products from which to share, collaborate, and accelerate knowledge creation.
- PEPFAR has had some success in external dissemination of PEPFAR knowledge, including establishing formal and informal mechanisms to share knowledge externally and contributing vast amounts of evidence and publications to the global knowledge base. Despite this, more progress is needed to develop routine formal mechanisms for knowledge exchange with partner country governments and other partners, increase the amount of PEPFAR data that is publicly available for use by researchers and evaluators, and track and measure PEPFAR's contribution to the global knowledge base.

Overall Conclusion

- PEPFAR has made progress in managing knowledge by developing systems for data creation and collection, streamlining program monitoring data, advancing PEPFAR's role and approach to evaluation and research, and utilizing a wide variety of mechanisms to transfer knowledge. Yet, like other entities involved in the global HIV/AIDS response, it struggles with creating, acquiring, and transferring the right knowledge, at the appropriate scale, and in a manner that facilitates use. PEPFAR has the potential to lead the global HIV/AIDS community in knowledge management by adopting a conceptual framework that articulates the vision, purposes, intended audiences, and goals of knowledge; how knowledge will be acquired, created, transferred, used, and disseminated to achieve these goals; and the complementary roles of program monitoring, evaluation, and research. PEPFAR has the opportunity to optimize program efficiency and effectiveness through an improved strategy that (1) streamlines and focuses knowledge creation within PEPFAR; (2) increases acquisition of knowledge external to PEPFAR; (3) improves the efficiency and effectiveness of knowledge transfer within and external to PEPFAR; and (4) institutionalizes the use of knowledge to improve the way work is accomplished.

Recommendations Presented in This Chapter

Recommendation 11-1: The Office of the U.S. Global AIDS Coordinator (OGAC) should develop a comprehensive knowledge management framework, including a program monitoring and evaluation strategy, a prioritized and targeted research portfolio, and systems for knowledge dissemination. This framework should adapt to emerging needs to assess PEPFAR's models of implementation and contribution to sustainable management of the HIV response in partner countries.

This knowledge management framework will require that PEPFAR implement and strategically allocate resources for the following:

A. To better document PEPFAR's progress and effectiveness, OGAC should refine its program monitoring and evaluation strategy to streamline reporting and to strategically coordinate a complementary portfolio of evaluation activities to assess outcomes and effects that are not captured well by program monitoring indicators. Efforts should support innovation in methodologies and measures where needed. Both monitoring and evaluation should be specifically matched to clearly articulated data sources, methods, and uses at each level of PEPFAR's implementation and oversight.

B. To contribute to filling critical knowledge gaps that impede effective and sustainable HIV programs, OGAC should continue to redefine permitted research within PEPFAR by developing a prioritized portfolio with articulated activities and methods. The planning and implementation process at the country and program level should inform and be informed by the research portfolio, which should focus on research that will improve the effectiveness, quality, and efficiency of PEPFAR-supported activities and will also contribute to the global knowledge base on implementation of HIV/AIDS programs.

C. To maximize the use of knowledge created within PEPFAR, OGAC should develop systems and processes for routine, active transfer and dissemination of knowledge both within and external to PEPFAR. As one component, OGAC should institute a data-sharing policy, developed through a consultative process. The policy should identify the data to be included and ensure that these stipulated data and results generated by PEPFAR or through PEPFAR-supported activities are made available in a timely manner to PEPFAR stakeholders, external evaluators, the research community, and other interested parties.

Further considerations for implementation of Recommendation 11-1A: Program monitoring and evaluation

- OGAC's current tiered program monitoring indicator reporting structure (illustrated in Figure 11-10) should be further streamlined to report upward only those indicators essential at each PEPFAR level:
  - Tier 1: A small set of core indicators, fewer than the current 25, to be reported to central HQ level. These data should be used to monitor performance across PEPFAR as a whole, for congressional reporting, and to document trends; as such these indicators should remain consistent over time. Whenever possible and appropriate, these indicators should be harmonized with existing global indicators and national indicators; therefore, some centrally reported indicators will reflect PEPFAR's contribution rather than aim to measure direct attribution.
  - Tier 2: A larger menu of indicators defined in OGAC guidance, from which a subset are selected for their applicability to country programs to be reported by implementing partners to the U.S. mission teams but not routinely reported to HQ. These data should be used to monitor the effectiveness of the in-country response and to support mutual accountability with partner countries and their citizens. These data could be considered for occasional centralized use to inform special studies or respond to congressional requests but aggregation and comparability across countries may be limited in this tier as all mission teams may not collect the same data.
  - Tier 3: Indicators selected by implementing partners to monitor and manage program implementation and effectiveness that are not routinely reported to mission teams. Implementing partners should select appropriate indicators defined in OGAC guidance and augment these with other indicators as needed for their programs. Implementing partners should work with mission teams in developing their program monitoring plans with selected indicators. Mission teams should provide oversight and technical assistance to ensure implementation of these plans and to promote local quality data collection, use, and mutual accountability. Although not routinely reported, some of these data could be considered for occasional country-level and centralized use.
  - OGAC should create mechanisms for implementing partners, mission teams, and agency headquarters to mutually contribute to a periodic review across all tiers of indicator development, applicability, and utility and to make modifications if necessary.
  - Tier 1 indicators should be harmonized whenever possible and appropriate with existing global indicators and national indicators. For indicators that are not routinely reported centrally (Tiers 2 and 3), country program planning should facilitate alignment of

indicator selection and data collection with partner country HIV monitoring and health information systems.

- OGAC should complement program monitoring with a unified evaluation portfolio that includes periodic program evaluation at the PEPFAR country program and implementing partner levels to assess process, progress, and outcomes as well as periodic impact evaluations at the country, multi-country, and headquarters levels.
    - OGAC evaluation guidance should provide information about prioritizing areas for evaluation, the types of evaluation questions, methodological guidance, potential study designs, template evaluation plans, examples of key outcomes, and how evaluation results should be used and disseminated. PEPFAR should support a range of appropriate methodologies for program evaluation, including mixed qualitative and quantitative methods, and should shift emphasis from probability designs to plausibility designs that provide valid evidence of impact.
        - To allow for some comparability across countries and programs, OGAC and HQ technical working groups should, with input from country teams, strategically plan and coordinate a subset of evaluations within programmatic areas that include (but are not limited to) a minimum set of centrally identified and defined outcome measures and methodologies.
        - Within PEPFAR-supported evaluation activities there should be an emphasis on the use of in-country local expertise to enhance capacity building for program evaluation and contribute to country ownership.
- For both program monitoring and evaluation OGAC should continue its work on defining and developing measures to assess progress in the currently under-measured areas of country ownership, sustainability, gender, policy, capacity building and technical assistance.

Further considerations for implementation of Recommendation 11-1B: Research

- OGAC should clearly define which activities and methodologies will be included under the umbrella of PEPFAR-supported research, as distinguished from program evaluation.
- OGAC should draw on input from implementing agencies, mission teams, partner countries, implementing partners, the Scientific Advisory Board, and other experts to identify and articulate research priorities and appropriate research methodologies. The research proposals and funding mechanisms should be designed to ensure that these priorities are met and that methodologies are applied through requests for applications and other investigator-driven research pro-

posals as well as through targeted solicitations of research in gap areas not met through open requests.

- Given PEPFAR's legislative and programmatic objectives to support research that assesses program quality, effectiveness, and population-based impact; optimizes service delivery; and contributes to the global evidence base on HIV/AIDS interventions and program implementation, at the time of this evaluation the committee identified the following gaps in PEPFAR's research activities:
    - Behavioral and structural interventions, especially in areas such as prevention, gender, nonclinical care and support, care and support for orphans and vulnerable children, and treatment retention and adherence. These research activities should employ appropriate methodologies and study designs, without being unduly limited to random assignment designs.
    - Costs, benefits, and feasibility of integrating gender-focused programs with clinical and community-based activities.
    - Health systems strengthening interventions across the World Health Organization building blocks, with a prioritized goal of determining setting- and system-specific feasibility, effectiveness, quality of services, and costs for innovative models.
- To contribute to country ownership, PEPFAR should facilitate in-country local participation and research capacity building through simplified, streamlined, and transparent application and review processes that encourage submissions from country-based implementing partners and researchers.

Further considerations for implementation of Recommendation 11-1C: Knowledge transfer and dissemination

- The knowledge created within PEPFAR that should be more widely documented and disseminated includes program monitoring data, financial data, research results, evaluation outcomes, best practices, and informal knowledge such as implementation experience, and lessons learned.
- To institutionalize internal and external knowledge transfer and learning, PEPFAR should develop appropriate systems and processes for the most needed types and scale of knowledge transfer. To achieve this, PEPFAR should draw on broad stakeholder input to assess the strengths and weaknesses in current processes and to identify needs and opportunities for improved knowledge transfer.
- PEPFAR should invest in innovative mechanisms and technology to facilitate knowledge transfer across partner countries and implementing partners. Mechanisms currently used successfully on a small scale and an ad hoc basis could be formally scaled up across PEPFAR.

OGAC should also look to other organizations with wide geographic reach and organizational complexity, such as multi-country PEPFAR implementing partners, other large global health initiatives, and global corporations, for models of successful knowledge transfer systems.

- OGAC should develop a policy for data sharing and transparency that facilitates timely access to PEPFAR-created knowledge for analysis and evaluation. The purpose of this policy would be to ensure that, within a purposefully and reasonably defined scope, specified program monitoring data and financial data, evaluation outcomes, and research data and results generated with PEPFAR support by contractors, grantees, mission teams, and U.S. Government (USG) agencies be made available to the public, research community, and other external stakeholders. OGAC and the PEPFAR implementing agencies should consult with both internal and external parties who would be affected by this policy to help identify the data that are most critical for external access and that can be reasonably subject to data-sharing requirements, as well as to help develop feasible mechanisms to implement a data- sharing policy.
    - For routinely collected financial and program monitoring data, a limited set of essential data should be identified and made available for external use in a timely way.
    - Evaluation and research reports and publications using data collected through PEPFAR-supported programs should be tracked and made available in a publicly accessible central repository. USG agencies with similar repositories can be considered as models.
    - For research data and other information that is expressly generated for new knowledge, the policy should respect time-bound exclusivity for the right to engage in the publication process, yet also ensure the timely availability of data, regardless of publication, for access and use by external evaluators and researchers. OGAC should look to USG agencies with similar research data policies as models.
    - In developing the policy and specifying the scope of data to be included, several key factors and potential constraints that can affect the implementation of the policy will need to be addressed. These include patient and client information confidentiality; the financial resources, personnel, and time needed to make data available; and issues of data ownership, especially in the context of increasing responsibility in partner countries and the provision of PEPFAR support through country systems or through activities and programs supported by multiple funding streams.